SO YOU WANT THE PERFECT BODY?

Chris Pelosi Gym Fitness Instructor & Personal Trainer

Library of Congress Control Number: 2016910654
ISBN: Hardcover   978-1-5144-9760-9
                 Softcover   978-1-5144-9759-3
                 eBook   978-1-5144-9758-6

Rev. date: 06/29/2016

SO YOU WANT THE PERFECT BODY?

NOTES FROM THE AUTHOR

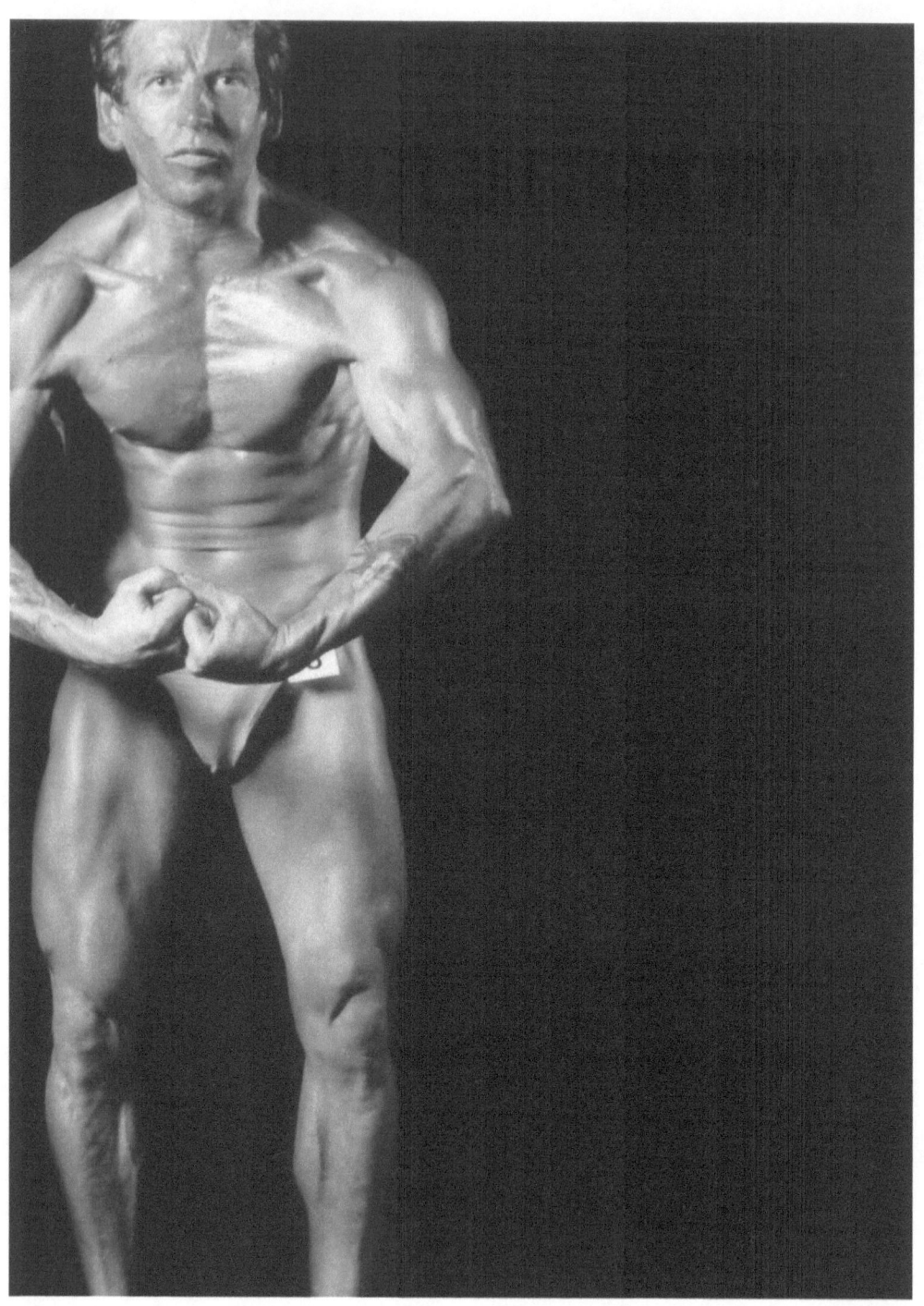

INTRODUCTION

This is a book dedicated to those who want to maintain a lifestyle in health and fitness.

I wrote this book in 2008 after successfully competing in state bodybuilding titles as a guide to others who may wish to benefit from my experience.

I have tried to compile all aspects of training into one easy concise manual for anyone wishing to maintain their body weight or improve the way they look.

I wish you all the best for the future and good luck!

STRETCHING

"Do stretches before you exercise a must"

Stretching is the most important part of your training cycle. It is at the start of a workout, so you prepare your muscles for a more strenuous exercise without tearing or damaging your muscles.

And should also be done at the end of your workout, to stop blood pooling in your muscles.

And also aids in the first step of recovery.

STRETCHES

BICEPS	With left arm straight out in front, use right hand to grasp fingers, bend left wrist and tense hold for 15 seconds and change hands.

TRICEPS	With left arm overhead bent at elbow and pointing down the centre of your back, bring right arm over grasp elbow and apply pulling pressure hold for 15 seconds and change arms.

DELTOIDS	Left arm across your chest using right arm with closed fist press behind elbow and pull towards chest and change arms.

PECS	With both hands behind back interlock fingers push back and up.

LATTS	Sitting on mat right leg straight and left leg bent at knee, and left foot on outside of right knee, twist upper body to the right, left arm braced in front of left knee, and apply pressure in twisting motion and hold, then change sides.

LATTS + ABBS	Sit on the floor mat with left leg, straight and right leg bent, with heal at your crutch, place left arm behind right leg and apply twisting pressure, and hold, then change sides. Also does Abbs.

QUADS	Stand tall on left leg while right leg is bent at the knee, from behind grasp foot and pull up into your glutes, you will feel stretching on your right thigh (quad) hold and release, change legs.

HAMSTRINGS	There is 2 ways to do this. Stand near a rail or beam about waist high, place one leg up on rail or beam while standing on other leg, straighten leg on rail and bend forward touching toes, apply slight pressure, hold and change legs.
	Or sit on floor mat with both legs straight out in front of you and lean forward with both hands trying to touch your toes.

CALVES	Standing 3 feet or 1 metre from a wall, place both hands on wall and bring one leg up to wall bent at knee while keeping other leg up to wall bent at knee while keeping other leg straight behind with heal on floor.

NOTE During stretches do not jerk or bounce- apply slight pressure only and hold for 15 seconds and release.

WEIGHT TRAINING EXERCISE

BEGINNERS

ABDOMINALS AND OBLIQUES	
TWIST	Broom stick over shoulders and twist from side to side from waist up.
SIDE BENDS	With dumbbell in each hand and feet shoulder width apart. Bend to one side, then bend to other side = 2 reps.
DECLINE SIT UPS	Place bench in elevated position legs over bar and come half way up. Squeeze abs and lower slowly.

CALVES	
STANDING CALF RAISE	Stand on 4 inch block with balls of feet, weight in one hand, use other hand for support and raise as high as you can go and lower heals down full stretch.
SEATED CALF RAISE	Sit on bench with leg extension on thighs, feet on block, then raise and lower heals.

QUADRICEPS	
(THIGHS) SQUATS	Raise bar to back of neck squat down till quads are horizontal and stand back up.
LEG EXTENSIONS	Sit on bench, feet under pads, raise and straighten legs tensing quads, lower slowly.

QUADRICEPS CONT.	
LUNGES	With weight in position for squats, step forward with one leg and back up, then other leg.

HAMSTRINGS	
LEG CURLS	Lay face down on bench, feet under pad, curl legs up tensing glutes and hamstrings.
STANDING LEG CURLS	Support yourself with one hand, place one leg behind pad and curl up tensing glutes and hamstring. Do required reps and change legs.

PECS	
BENCH PRESS	Lay on bench with a wide grip on bar, lift bar up and lower to pecs and press bar up tensing pecs.
FLY'S	Laying on bench (chest up), swing dumbbells up with elbows slightly bent, lower dumbbells out and down, and keeping elbows bent raise back up.
DIPS	Grasp handles with legs bent and crossed lower then raise tensing pecs.
DUMBBELL INCLINE	Laying on bench swing dumbbells up above head and touch dumbbells together, then lower and raise tensing pecs.

LATTS	
BENT OVER ROW	Bend over with legs slightly bent and wide grip pull bar to pecs and lower.

LATTS CONT.	
LATT PULL DOWN BEHIND NECK	Sit on bench, grip bar wider than shoulder width, pull bar behind neck tensing latts, then raise bar backup stretching latts.
DUMBBELL PULLOVER	With shoulders and head on bench grip dumbbell hold above head and lower behind stretching ribs and latts and raise back up.
DUMBBELL ROW	With one knee and hand on bench bend over with dumbbell in one hand and pull up to chest tensing latts then lower.
CABLE ROW	Sit on bench with close grip pull handle to abbs tensing latts and release slowly.
HIGH CABLE ROW	Sit on bench reach up and grip bar, close grip, pull handle to pecs tensing latts and let back up stretching latts.

DELTOIDS	
PRESS BEHIND NECK	With a grip slightly wider than shoulder width raise bar over head and lower to base of neck and press back up tensing delts.
UPRIGHT ROW	Grip bar thumb width grip, stand up and pull bar to chin with elbows high and lower.
SIDE LATTERALS	Grip dumbbell in front, raise out and up lower slowly.
FRONT RAISE	Grip dumbbells in front, raise out and up lower slowly.
BENT OVER LATTERALS	With dumbbells in each hand, elbows bent, bend over and raise dumbbells out and up lower slowly.

TRAPEZIUS	
SHRUGS	With dumbbell in each hand try to touch ears with deltoids, starting from front, roll dumbbells behind and lower.

BICEPS	
BARBELL CURLS	Grip barbell with shoulder width grip, curl bar to shoulders tensing biceps, lower slowly.

INCLINE DUMB-BELL CURLS	Seated on incline bench with dumbbell in each hand curl to shoulders tensing biceps, lower slowly.

CABLE CURLS	Support yourself on bench while standing grip bar and curl to shoulders and lower slowly.

CONCENTRA-TION CURLS	Sit on bench and bend over with dumbbell in hand, support elbow on thigh and curl to shoulder tensing biceps lower slowly.

TRICEPS	
TRICEPS PUSHDOWNS	Standing over bench grip latt bar and pull down till arms are at 90°, push down to arms length and release slowly.

LYING TRICEPS PRESS	Lay on bench grip bar shoulder width grip, lift bar off rack keeping elbows high, lower to forehead and press back up tensing triceps.

DUMBBELL KICKBACKS	Supporting with one hand on bench with knee on bench hold arm at 90 degrees with dumbbell and kick back to straighten arm and lower slowly.

WEIGHT TRAINING EXERCISE

ADVANCED EXTRA'S

ABDOMINALS	
HANGING LEG RAISE ABDOMINAL CRUNCH	On a beam over your head, grasp beam legs bent, curl body while raising knees to chest tensing abbs lowers slowly.

QUADRICEPS	
DEAD LIFTS	With heavy weights on barbell grip bar one hand, under and one hand over, feet shoulder width apart, keeping back straight stand up and lower.

PECS	
REVERSE BENCH PRESS	With 2 spotters one each side, holding a weight each, lay on bench, lift bar off rack and up. Spotters place a heavy weight each end and lower over 6 seconds, take weights off and repeat 6 times, once a month.

LATTS	
LATTS PULLDOWNS FRONT OF NECK	With wide grip, pull bar to front of neck and release.
REVERSE GRIP BENT OVER ROWS	With shoulder width grip, grasp bar underhand grip feet shoulder width apart, bend over keeping back straight pull barbell to abbs tensing latts and lower.

LATTS CONT.	
HANGING LATTS PULLUPS	While hanging from beam with wide grip pull up till beam is at back of neck, lower slowly.

BICEPS	
PREACHER CURLS	Sit on bench facing preacher bench, grip barbell shoulder width grip and curl bar to deltoids and lower slowly.

TRICEPS	
TRICEPS EXTENSIONS	With dumbbell in each hand swing them above head with elbows firm, lower dumbbells till arms are bent at 90 degrees and press backup tensing triceps.

NOTES

ISOMETRICS

Isometrics is another way of building a strong Physique without the use of weights or machines, using only your body and body parts eg. hands, arms and legs to apply resistance and force to strengthen your muscles and tone up. Bigger gains in strength and definition. (5 minutes a day.)

FOREARMS	Clasp and interlock fingers of each hand together and twist hands in opposite directions at 8 second intervals of pressure hold and release.
BICEPS AND TRICEPS	Standing up with left hand bent at elbow and palm facing upwards place clenched fist of right hand on top of your palm and apply pressure = max up and down, hold for 8 seconds and change hands.
LATTS	Again in a hugging embrace grasp left wrist with right hand and pull stretching forward and hold.
DELTOIDS	Stand in a doorway and place backs of hands against door frame and push outwards, hold for 8 seconds and release.
QUADS + HAMSTRING	In a sitting position on edge of chair place one foot over other foot with bent legs at 90° push and pull for 8 seconds and change legs.
CALVES	In a sitting position bend knees out to the side and place soles of feet together and push against each other, hold and release.

POSING

Once you have finished your weight training program, you may want to enter competitions and gain that elusive trophy. Entry to competitions can be found at most good gyms, they will happy to point you in the right direction.

YOU WILL NEED:
- posing costume
- a tanning solution used only for contests
- 1 spray can of cooking oil
- 1 tape of 60 seconds of music for your routine
- *smile*

THERE ARE 10 COMPULSORY POSES YOU WILL PERFORM ON STAGE.
1. Abdominal with thighs
2. Double biceps front
3. latt spread front
4. side chest pose (left)
5. side chest pose (right)
6. double biceps with a calf rear
7. latt spread with other calf rear
8. tricep left side
9. tricep right side
10. your most muscular pose

Combine all of these poses and hold each one for 15 seconds.

PROTEIN

FIRST CLASS PROTEIN
Egg, chicken, meat, fish, milk, cheese and yoghurt.

First class proteins must be consumed at every meal when body building, it is recommended that you consume 2-2½ grams of protein per kilo of body weight each day, approx 150 grams a day, try to eat 40 grams per meal.

EG. Breakfast, lunch, dinner and supper. Spacing your 4 meals and 3 protein drinks a day, it is quality not quantity that matters. By eating small but quality meals, your stomach will stay flat. Your snacks between meals will consist of protein drinks, IE, milk and egg-whites.

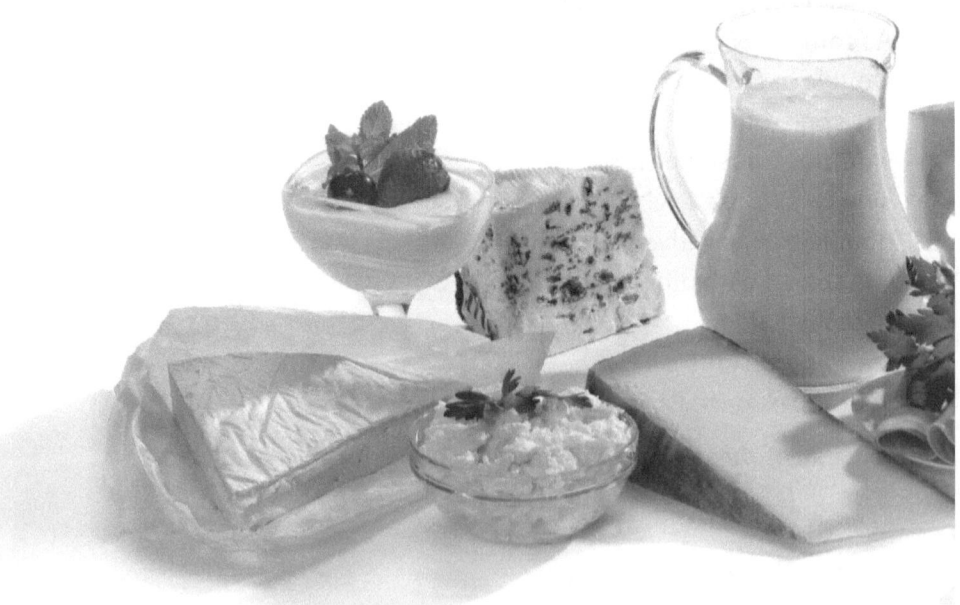

PROTEIN SHAKES

300ml of skim milk, or tone milk and 4 egg-whites (approx 300 grams) mixed in a shaker and consume between meals, with an apple, orange or banana, between breakfast and lunch, lunch and dinner, dinner and supper.

FOOD	AMOUNT	PROTEIN (grams)
skim milk	1 litre	40
cheese	30g	6
yoghurt	1 litre	40
egg-whites	1	6
chicken breast	1	40
tuna	185g tin	40
fish-fillet		40
steak t-bone		40
low fat mince	250g	40

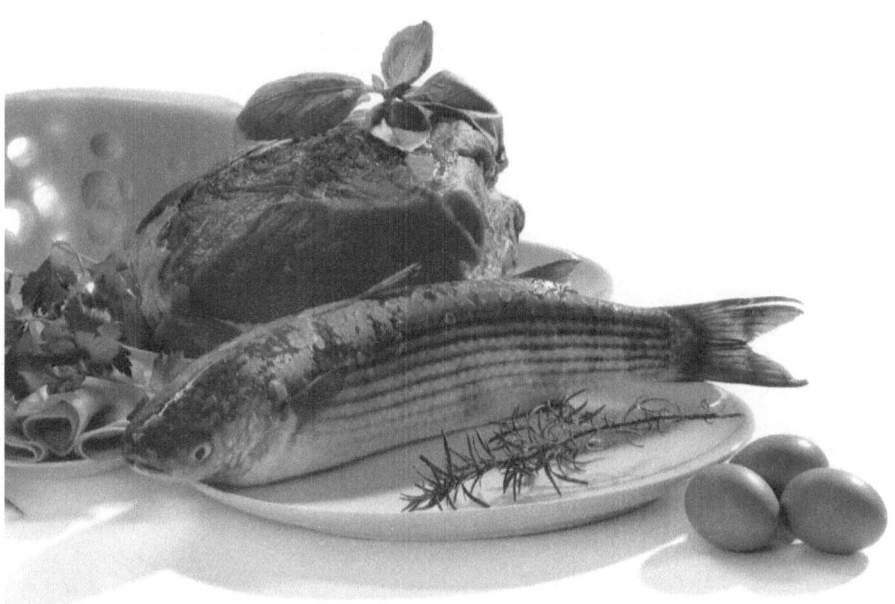

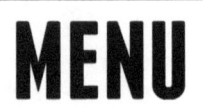

MENU

	MONDAY	TUESDAY	WEDNESDAY
BREAKFAST	150ml egg white, scramble,1 toast, 50g cereal, protein shake	150ml egg white, anyway,1 toast, 50g cereal, protein shake	150ml egg white, scramble,1 toast, 50g cereal, protein shake
	You may alternate baked beans for egg whites.		

SNACK	protein shake, piece of fruit

LUNCH	185g can of tuna/salad with either rice or pasta and 2 slices of

SNACK	Protein shake, piece of fruit

DINNER	steak, 3 veg	chicken salad	fish salad
	Tea, coffee, skim milk or tone milk.		

SUPPER	Protein shake, tin fruit and low fat yoghurt.

! Use a non-stick fry pan for cooking eggs and meat. You may use olive oil, as it is 77% digestible. The other 23% you will burn off with your workout, for cooking use 1 tbsp of olive oil. Try to take a brisk walk for 40 minutes non stop 3 times a week.

THURSDAY	FRIDAY	SATURDAY	SUNDAY
150ml egg white, anyway,1 toast, 50g cereal, protein shake	150ml egg white, scramble,1 toast, 50g cereal, protein shake	150ml egg white, anyway,1 toast, 50g cereal, protein shake	150ml egg white, scramble,1 toast, 50g cereal, protein shake
multi-grain bread. Tea or coffee.			
steak, 3 veg	chicken salad	fish salad	roast, 3 veg

WEIGHT TRAINING CYCLES

STAGE 1

<table>
<tr><td align="center">MONDAY   WEDNESDAY   FRIDAY
ABBS - PECS - LATTS - TRAPS - CALVES</td><td align="center">TUESDAY   THURSDAY
DELTOIDS - BICEPS - TRICEPS - QUADRICEPS</td></tr>
</table>

6 week training cycle - 5 weeks training and 1 week rest.
In the 3rd week for 1 week only you will change your program to a circuit.

			WEEK	**1**			**2**			**3**			**4**			**5**		
		Set	**reps**	M	W	F	M	W	F	M	W	F	M	W	F	M	W	F
	twists		50							circuit								
ABBS	decline sit ups	2x	max															
	sidebends		50															
PECS	bench press	2x	12															
LATTS	bent over row	2x	12															
TRAPS	dumbbell shrugs	2 x	12															
CALVES	standing calf raise	2x	12															

				T T		**T T**		**T T**		**T T**		**T T**	
DELTOID	press behind neck	2x	12										
BICEPS	barbell curls	2x	12										
TRICEPS	tri-pushdown	2x	12										
QUADS	squats	2x	8										

STAGE 2

<table>
<tr><td>**MONDAY   WEDNESDAY   FRIDAY**
ABBS - PECS - LATTS - TRAPS - CALVES</td><td>**TUESDAY   THURSDAY**
DELTOIDS - BICEPS - TRICEPS - QUADRICEPS</td></tr>
</table>

			WEEK	1	2	3	4	5
		Set	**reps**	M W F	M W F	M W F	M W F	M W F
ABBS	twists		100			circuit		
	decline sit ups	3x	max					
	sidebends		50					
PECS	bench press	3x	10					
	flyes	2x	8					
LATTS	bent over row	3x	10					
	pulldown behind neck	2x	8					
TRAPS	dumbbell shrugs	3x	10					
CALVES	standing calf raise	3x	max					

				T T	T T	T T	T T	T T
DELTOID	press behind neck	3x	10					
	side/laterals	2x	6					
BICEPS	barbell curls	3x	10					
	incline curls	2x	8					
TRICEPS	tri-pushdown	3x	10					
	lying tri-press	2x	8					
QUADS	squats	3x	8					
	leg extension	2x	12					

STAGE 3 & 4 (opposite page)

<table>
<tr><td>**MONDAY   WEDNESDAY   FRIDAY**
ABBS - PECS - LATTS - TRAPS - CALVES</td><td>**TUESDAY   THURSDAY**
DELTOIDS - BICEPS - TRICEPS - QUADRICEPS - HAMSTRINGS</td></tr>
</table>

		Set	reps	WEEK 1 M W F	2 M W F	3 M W F	4 M W F	5 M W F
ABBS	twists		100			circuit		
	decline sit ups	3x	max					
	sidebends		50					
PECS	bench press	3x	8					
	flyes	3x	6					
LATTS	bent over row	3x	8					
	pulldown behind neck	2x	10					
TRAPS	dumbbell shrugs	3x	10					
CALVES	standing calf raise	3x	max					

		Set	reps	T T	T T	T T	T T	T T
DELTOID	press behind neck	3x	8					
	side/laterals	2x	8					
	bentover laterals	2x	8					
BICEPS	barbell curls	3x	8					
	incline curls	3x	8					
TRICEPS	tri-pushdown	3x	6					
	lying tri-press	3x	6					
QUADS	squats	3x	8					
	leg extension	3x	10					
HAM-STRINGS	lying leg curls	2x	8					

		Set	reps	WEEK 1 M W F	2 M W F	3 M W F	4 M W F	5 M W F
ABBS	twists		100			circuit		
	decline sit ups	4x	max					
	sidebends		50					
PECS	bench press	4x	8.8.6.4					
	flyes	3x	10					
	pullovers	3x	10					
LATTS	bent over row	4x	8.8.6.4					
	latt pulldown behind neck	3x	10					
	dumbbell row	2x	12					
TRAPS	dumbbell shrugs	4x	8.8.6.4					
CALVES	standing calf raise	4x	max					
	seated calf raise	2x	max					

		Set	reps	T T	T T	T T	T T	T T
DELTOID	press behind neck	4x	8.8.6.4					
	side/laterals	3x	8					
	bentover laterals	3x	8					
BICEPS	barbell curls	4x	8.8.6.4					
	incline curls	3x	6					
	cable curls	2x	6					
TRICEPS	tri-pushdown	4x	8.8.6.4					
	lying tri-press	3x	6					
	dumbbell kick-backs	2x	8					
QUADS	squats	4x	8.8.6.4					
	leg extension	3x	12					
	dead lifts	2x	12					
HAM-STRINGS	lying leg curls	3x	8					

STAGE 5

			WEEK		1			2			3			4			5		
		Set	reps		M	W	F	M	W	F	M	W	F	M	W	F	M	W	F
ABBS	twists		100								circuit								
	decline sit ups	4x	max																
	sidebends		50																
	hanging leg raises	2x	max																
PECS	bench press	4x	6.6.4.2																
	flyes	4x	6																
	pullovers	4x	8																
	dips	2x	max																
LATTS	bent over row	4x	6.6.4.2																
	latt pulldown behind neck	4x	6																
	dumbbell row	4x	8																
	cable row	4x	8																
TRAPS	dumbbell shrugs	4x	6																
CALVES	standing calf raise	4x	max																
	seated calf raise	2x	max																

		Set	reps	WEEK 1 T T	2 T T	3 T T	4 T T	5 T T
DELTOID	press behind neck	4x	6.6.4.2			circuit		
	side/laterals	4x	6					
	bentover laterals	4x	6					
	upright row	4x	6					
BICEPS	barbell curls	4x	6					
	incline curls	4x	6					
	cable curls	4x	6					
	preacher curls	4x	6.6.3.2					
TRICEPS	tri-pushdown	4x	6.6.3.2					
	lying tri-press	4x	6.6.3.2					
	dumbbell kick-backs	4x	6.6.4.2					
	tricep extension	4x	6.6.4.2					
QUADS	squats	4x	6.6.4.2					
	leg extension	4x	8					
	lunges	4x	6					
	dead lifts	4x	6.4.3.2					
HAM-STRINGS	lying leg curls	4x	6.4.3.2					
	standing leg curls	3x	5.4.3.2					

SO YOU WANT THE PERFECT BODY?

The most important part of this program is -
diet, exercise, sleep, relaxation + recovery.

Firstly with this diet you will maintain, and even gain lean muscle mass while reducing body-fat.

Lean meat - skinless chicken, fish grilled, meat that is either stewed or roasted is the best and low in fat.

When you miss meals your body goes into starvation mode, because it doesn't know when the next meal is coming, so it stores body-fat, and you put on unwanted weight.

By doing a wide range of exercises, and eating small meals 5 times a day the bodies metabolism speeds up and burns body-fat.

When you begin your exercise always warm-up first, to prepare your body for more strenuous exercise.

It takes 20 minutes with elevated Heart rate and exercise eg: Aerobics, before you start to burn body-fat. So if you exercise for 40 minutes, then you have burnt off 20 minutes of body-fat.

If you stop you have to start all over again, so try to go for a brisk walk for 40 minutes non-stop, 3-4 times a week, walking is the best and safest way to start.

PROTEIN maintains and is the building block for lean muscle growth.

Each meal should consist of:

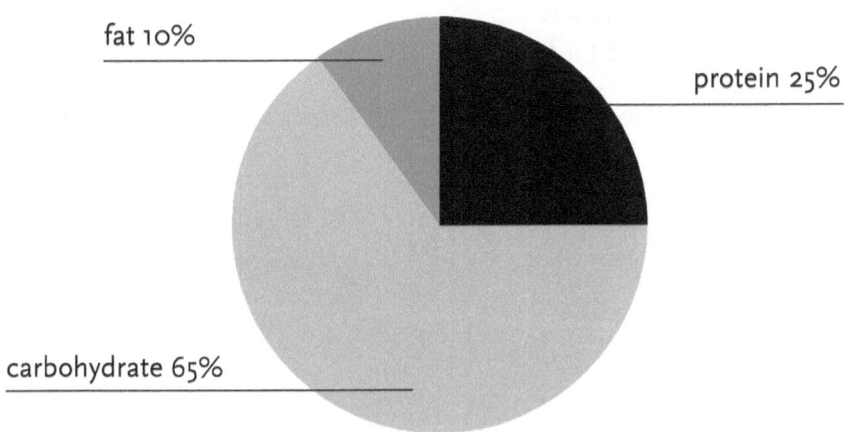

fat 10%

protein 25%

carbohydrate 65%

Your food even low fat and healthy still has fat - don't worry it's in there.

Egg white is natures most purest form of protein and rich in vitamins.

Meat, chicken, fish, cheese, milk and egg whites are all first class proteins.

Fatty foods are a very good source of energy, but very difficult to burn off.

Eg: cakes, biscuits, ice-cream, chocolates and fatty meats should be avoided.

The diet in this book is ideal for losing up to 1-kg of body fat per week while maintaining lean muscle growth, depending on the exercises you do.

Carbohydrates, potatoes, pasta, rice and oats etc are the best forms of energy, and should be consumed with breakfast, lunch and dinner that is energy for your workouts.

In 3 months on this diet combined with Isometrics and weight training, I went from a very slim 55kg to a medium build of 67kg and have maintained my physique for 10 years.

This program is a lifestyle, now at the age of 50, my body is still in the best condition.

Once you have done this program you may wish to vary your weights to build certain areas of your body.

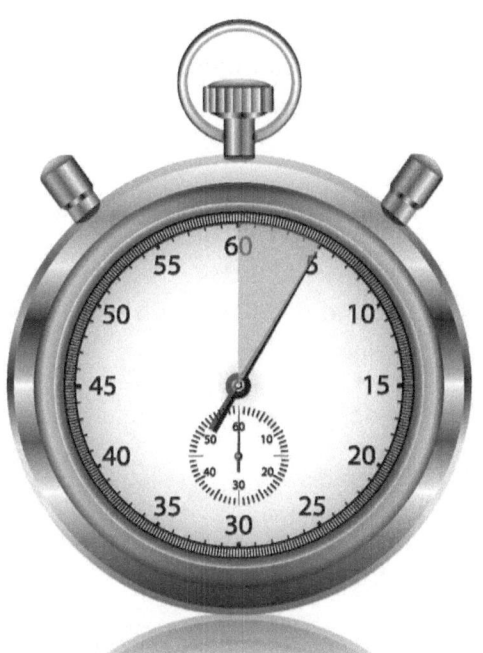

ISOMETRICS is another way of using your body, to tone and enhance your body, it is very efficient for toning and building those problem areas.

You can do them anywhere and anyway you like, you choose what part you want to perfect and exercise that part.

But it is better to do all of your body, just 5 minutes a day, twice a day.

From the very first time that you try Isometrics you will feel the muscles reacting against each other, watch them grow and tone up quite quickly. If you are doing weight training and you miss a workout, don't stress, do isometrics.

When you combine Isometrics with weight training it builds striations through your muscles, creating the exceptional body.

WEIGHT TRAINING when commencing a weight training regime as a beginner, pick a weight preferable something you can lift around 15 times in all exercises.

It is best to start light and build up gradually. Try to add 1-1¼ kg a week on all exercises.

With "bench - latts - squats and dead-lifts" you may increase up to 5 kg a week depending on how hard you train.

You should just be able to do the required reps in each set.

If you can do it easily, add more weight.

You will see yourself getting stronger and growing each time you workout.

After 3 weeks, you will start to see results, so encourage yourself to keep on with the training, as it takes around 3 weeks to develop a habit out of it.

If you are slim, you will start to add body bulk as you eat more and workout harder, lifting heavier weights.

If you are small you have to workout just the same, and eat more protein to build on your small frame.

If you are over weight, you will lose body fat while toning your body. Following this program the excess weight will fall off quite quickly, and your body mass eg muscle will stand out giving you that body you desire.

It's gradual, but a very effective way to get into shape and look good and feel proud of your body.

This program is beneficial for all body types.

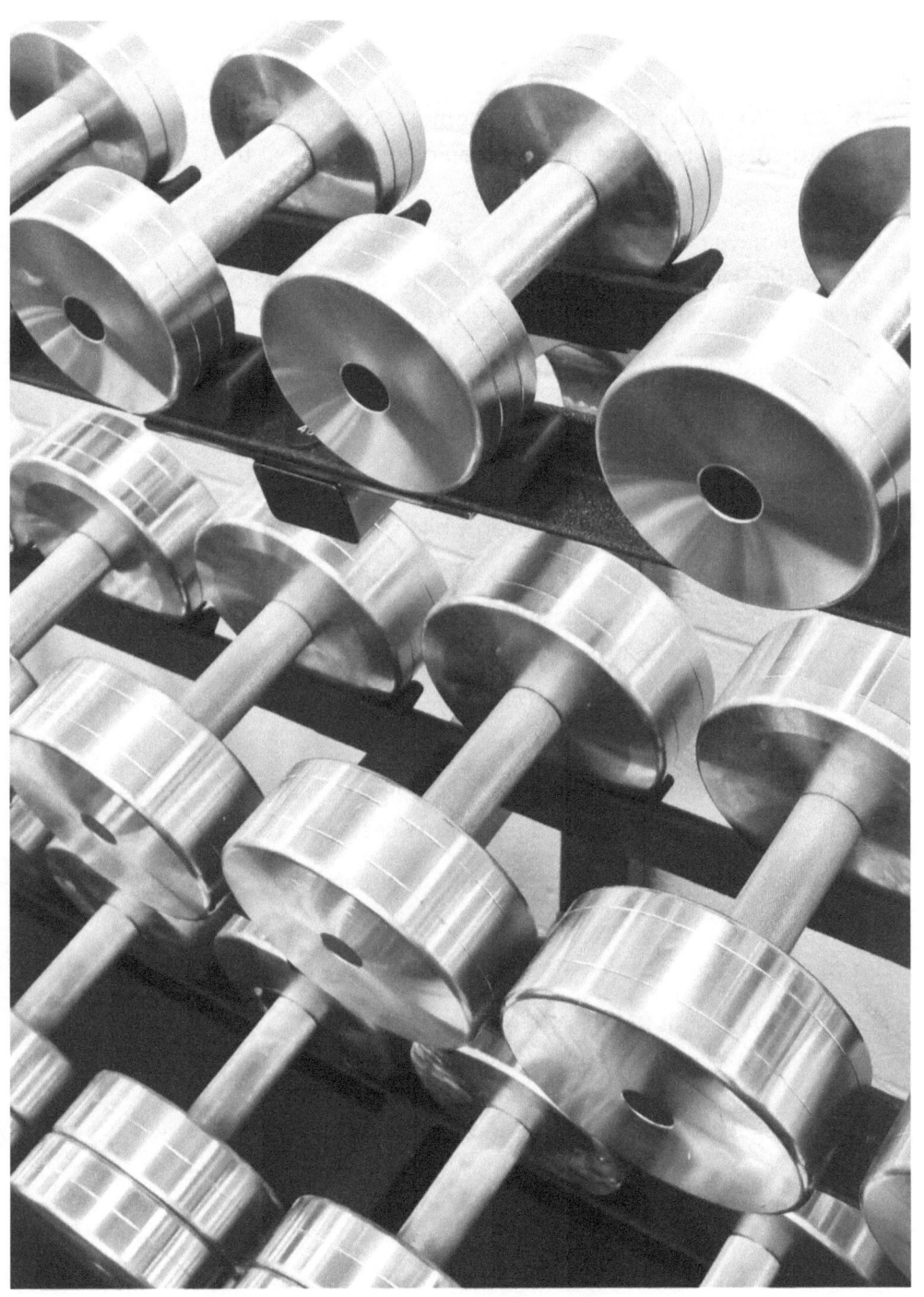

POSING when preparing for a contest you must have all the ingredients I have mentioned in the Posing section at the front of this book.

You will have to shave or wax your whole body.
Apply the tan liberally and have someone spray you with cooking oil.
The tan will wash off with soap and water.

A big smile and you are ready for competition.

You will need to have a routine.
eg. other slow moves and steps while flexing, to show the judges your best physique.
While on stage stay flexed all over, while sucking your stomach in.

The judges will ask for a pose, which you will do, but when they say relax DON'T, stay flexed in a relaxed position.
You will do this with other body builders on stage.

Then you will perform 1 at a time, to your own routine and your 10 poses, while your music plays for 60 seconds.

On stage you will see nothing but bright lights, and a cross on the floor, that's the point where the judges get the best look at you.

You will perform in the morning with other competitors, and then at night by yourself.

You may choose not to compete, you may just want the perfect body.

I hope you get out of this program what I have.
I wish you well in your endeavour to change your lifestyle.
You will be in control of your health, physical well-being and psychological state of mind, with the new you.

"I wish you well".

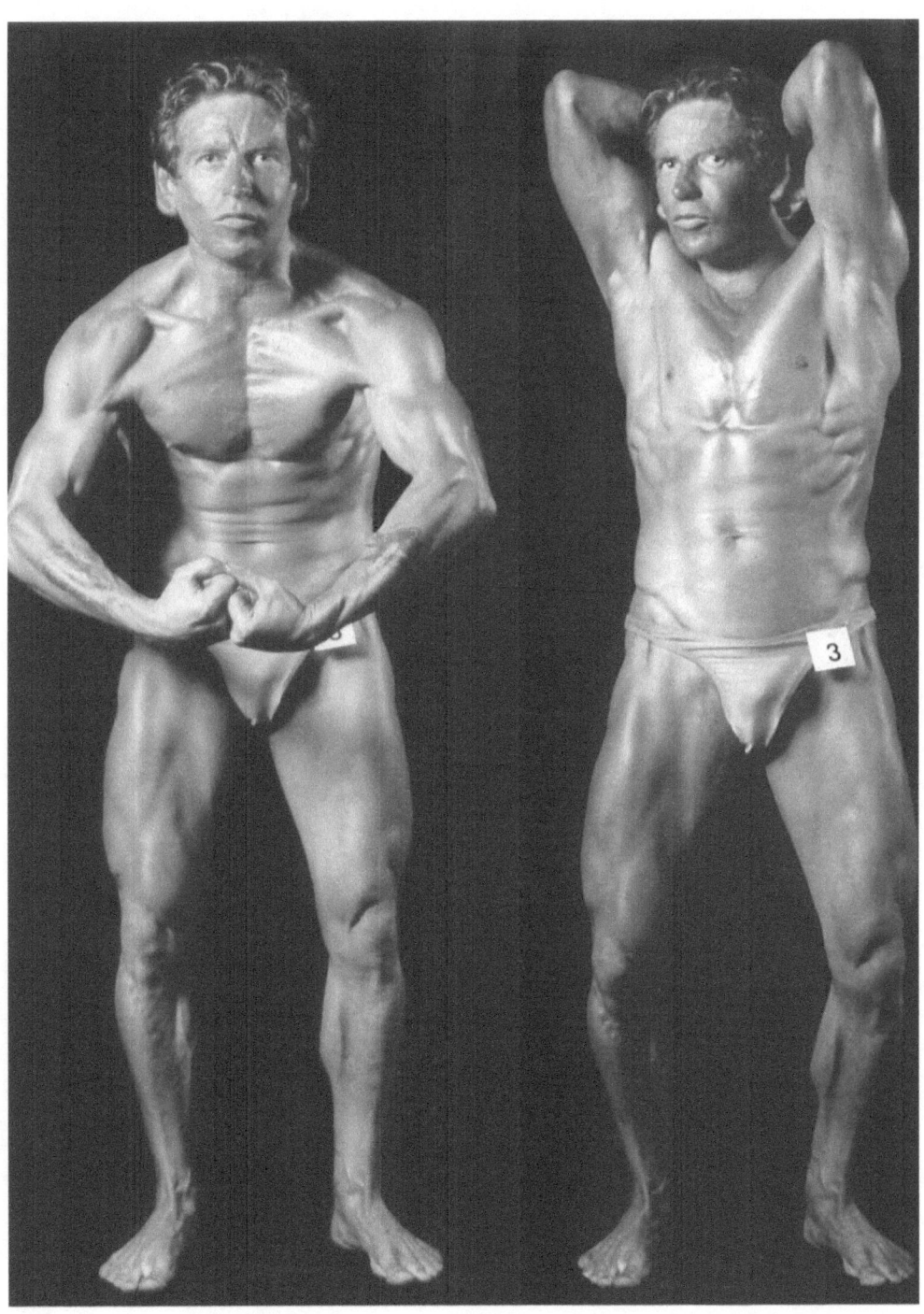

NOTES

NOTES

NOTES

NOTES

NOTES

NOTES

NOTES

NOTES

NOTES

NOTES

NOTES

NOTES